Healthy Habits

Mindful Eating for Optimal Nutrition

Table of Contents

Chapter 1. Introduction

Experience the invigorating journey towards a healthier lifestyle with our Special Report: "Healthy Habits: Mindful Eating for Optimal Nutrition". This expertly-crafted guide is not only a delight to explore but also a gentle nudge in the direction of transforming your relationship with food. As you navigate through its pages, you'll discover the compelling science behind mindful eating, alongside practical and easy-to-follow strategies that harness the power of focused attention and savouring. Unearth a treasure trove of valuable nuggets about nutrition, healthy food choices, and maintaining a balanced diet, woven into an engaging tapestry of appetizing recipes, smart shopping advice, and fitness tips. Make that crucial step towards a happier, healthier self today with this indispensable Special Report that promises not just information, but a transformative experience. So come, let us embark on this exciting venture towards mindful eating and optimal nutrition. It's time to turn the page towards better health and a vibrant life, one sustained bite at a time!

Chapter 2. The Power of Mindful Eating

We've all been there: finishing a meal and then barely remembering the textures and flavors that we've consumed. This often happens because we are distracted, either by the television, our smartphones, or even our wandering thoughts. But what if there was a better way to eat whereby we become completely present in the moment and can fully appreciate each mouthful? This is where mindful eating comes into play, a practice that is gaining worldwide attention for its myriad health benefits, both physically and psychologically.

2.1. The Basic Principles of Mindful Eating

Mindful eating is the art of consuming food with attention, intention, and mindfulness. It involves paying full attention to the experience of eating and drinking, both inside and outside the body. We pay attention to the colors, smells, textures, flavors, temperatures, and even the sounds of our food. We also pay attention to the experience of our body, where we notice hunger and fullness, and the liking or disliking of food.

1. Engage your senses: Experience the colors, textures, and smells of your food. Invite yourself to explore, savor and taste, being aware of each bite from beginning to end.

2. Savor the moment: Enjoy eating and respect the pace of your food, without rushing to finish your meal.

3. Be present: Eat with full consciousness and without distractions like TV or smartphones.

4. Be grateful: Appreciate the journey your food has taken to get to your plate.

2.2. Mindful Eating versus Mindless Eating

In contrast, mindless eating is when we eat without paying full attention to what, and how much, we are eating. Such eating habits often lead to overeating and ignoring our body's signals of fullness. Mindful eating helps to rebalance our relationship with food, helping us to eat less and enjoy food more.

2.3. The Remarkable Benefits of Mindful Eating

Chapter 3. Improved Digestion

When we eat mindfully, we chew slowly, aiding the process of digestion. Digestion begins in the mouth with the action of enzymes in saliva breaking down carbohydrates. By eating slowly, we ensure our food is well-digested, leading to better nutrient absorption.

Chapter 4. Reduction in Overeating

Mindful eating encourages you to pay heed to your body's hunger and fullness cues, which helps reduce bouts of overeating. When we savour every bite, we are more likely to stop eating when we feel comfortable and satisfied.

Chapter 5. Weight Management

Studies have shown that practicing mindful eating can be a useful tool in weight management. Mindful eating can enhance the pleasure of eating while also making people feel more satisfied after a meal.

Chapter 6. Relationship with Food

Mindful eating can transform your relationship with food, allowing you to enjoy your meals more and to recognize the difference between emotional hunger and physical hunger.

6.1. Techniques for Mindful Eating

Mindful eating requires a practice-based approach, and mastering it involves the body, mind and even our emotions. Here are a few techniques that you can incorporate into your daily regimen:

1. Start with small bites: Begin each meal with small bites and savour each one.

2. Chew thoroughly: Chew your food slowly and thoroughly, letting the flavours saturate your senses.

3. Put away distractions: Clear away any distractions like TV, books, or smartphones when you eat.

4. Eat slowly: Take time over your meal, don't rush. Remember, it's not a race.

5. Listen to your body: Learn to respond to hunger and fullness queues. Eat when you're hungry and stop when you're full.

=== Incorporating mindful eating into our day-to-day lives can completely transform our relationship with food. You can eat and still lose weight, improve your digestion, cope with food-related issues, and overall, feel healthier and happier. Mindful eating is not just about making healthier food choices; it's about recognising and honoring your body's needs without judgement. It empowers you to create a balanced and healthy approach to eating. Every meal then becomes an opportunity to nourish your body and mind.

Chapter 7. Endnote

Achieving mindfulness while eating involves fostering a new relationship with food. It's about making food a friend, not a foe, and embracing an attitude of moderation rather than deprivation. We learn to pay attention, to slow down, savor and enjoy our food. Gradually, these mindful practices become a part of who we are, rather than something we 'do'. And in this process of awakening our senses, we open ourselves to an even more richly satisfying way of eating, and living.

Chapter 8. Unpacking the Basics of Nutrition

Understanding the essence of nutrition is the first essential step in our mindful journey towards good health. As we delve into the intriguing world of nutrients, we'll uncover the vital role they play in providing us energy, supporting growth, and maintaining life.

8.1. Macronutrients

Macronutrients refer to the nutrients that our bodies need in large quantities, namely carbs, proteins, and fats.

Carbohydrates primarily serve as the body's main source of energy. They can be classified into simple (sugar) and complex (starch and fiber).

While simple carbohydrates provide quick energy, complex carbohydrates, such as whole grains and legumes, ensure a sustained energy release. They also deliver fiber, aiding in digestion and contributing to feelings of satiety, thus helping to support effective weight management.

Proteins construct, maintain, and repair our body tissues, cells, and organs. They also play a pivotal role in producing hormones and enzymes. Animal sources like meat, poultry, fish, eggs, and dairy, are rich protein sources, as are plant-based alternatives like beans, lentils, and nuts.

Fats are quite often misunderstood and associated solely with weight gain and health problems. However, they're a vital energy source and support cell growth while also helping protect our organs. Omega-3 and omega-6 fatty acids, both forms of unsaturated fats, are essential as our body cannot produce them. Foods such as fish, avocados, and nuts are excellent sources of these essential fats.

8.2. Micronutrients

Unlike the former, micronutrients are vital minerals and vitamins needed by our body in smaller amounts, but are indispensable for proper bodily function.

Vitamins are organic compounds vital for warding off diseases and staying healthy. Each vitamin has a particular role in the body. For example, Vitamin C can boost the immune system, Vitamin A aids in vision, and various B vitamins foster cell health.

Likewise, *Minerals* like calcium, potassium, and iron are essential for body functions. Calcium aids in bone health, potassium maintains fluid balance, and iron is critical for red blood cells that transport oxygen around our body.

8.3. Achieving a Balanced Diet

Having touched upon the basics of essential nutrients, let's look at how one can cultivate a balanced diet using these powerful components. A balanced diet should be our goal as it provides varied nutrients from food in the right proportions, promoting optimal health.

First and foremost, focus on incorporating a variety of foods into your meals. A rich and diverse diet ensures your body gets an assortment of necessary nutrients.

Including an adequate amount of protein, such as lean meats, eggs, or lentils, ensures that our bodies have the necessary building blocks to repair and renew cells and tissues.

Next, prioritizing complex carbohydrates, such as brown rice, whole grains, or fruits, will provide a steady release of energy throughout the day.

Healthy fats, including omega-3s from fish, monounsaturated fats from olive oil or avocados, and reducing the intake of saturated and trans fats, assist in supporting overall wellbeing.

Incorporating an abundance of fruits and vegetables is another cornerstone for a balanced diet. They're packed with vitamins, minerals, and antioxidants while being low in calories.

Finally, staying hydrated is just as crucial as the food you eat. Dehydration can lead to a series of health complications, from fatigue and headaches, to more serious issues like kidney and heart problems.

8.4. Understanding Food Labels

Wherever you are on your nutrition journey, knowing how to read and interpret food labels can arm you with the information you need to make healthy choices. Labels typically provide valuable information on calories, serving sizes, nutrients, and ingredients. Always seek foods that contain less added sugars, sodium, unhealthy fats, and opt for those higher in dietary fiber, vitamins, and minerals.

8.5. The Impact of Over- and Under-Nutrition

Over-nutrition and under-nutrition pose significant health risks. Over-nutrition, typically due to overeating nutrient-poor, high-calorie foods, can lead to overweight and obesity, escalating the risk of chronic diseases. Indeed, a balanced diet and regular physical activity can help maintain a healthy weight.

On the other hand, under-nutrition, the outcome of an insufficient intake of essential nutrients, leads to malnutrition. This can cause a host of health problems, from stunted growth in children, to weakened immune systems, and even impaired brain development.

8.6. The Role of Nutrient Timing

Finally, while what we eat is paramount, when we consume our meals also impacts our nutrition and health. Regular, balanced meals and snacks throughout the day can stabilize our blood glucose level, preventing energy peaks and troughs. Simultaneously, knowing when to hydrate, especially around physical activity, can significantly influence our performance and recovery.

Takeaway: Nutrition is an exciting yet complex world. Understanding it allows us to make informed food decisions, steer clear of dietary pitfalls, and nurture our bodies with the care they deserve. Providing ourselves not just with what's tasty, but what's nutritionally rich, equips us in leading a healthier, more vibrant life.

Chapter 9. Aligning Your Food Choices with Your Health Goals

Our journey to optimal nutrition and mindful eating begins by aligning our food choices with our health goals. This might sound like a daunting task, but breaking it down into manageable steps will simplify the process and make the journey more enjoyable and meaningful.

9.1. Understanding Your Health Goals

First, let's delve into understanding your health goals. These could range from losing weight, building muscle, controlling sugar intake for diabetes, or just maintaining a healthy lifestyle. It is important to pinpoint these objectives, as they will inform your food selections. Discuss with healthcare professionals, do some research, understand your body, and make informed decisions.

9.2. Making Informed Food Choices

Once your goals are established, make a conscious effort to select foods that will contribute towards those goals. This may involve reducing intake of processed foods, increasing fruits and vegetables, substituting unhealthy snacks with healthier alternatives, or modulating portion sizes.

Pay attention to food labels. Understand the macronutrient and micronutrient contents. It's helpful to familiarize yourself with what constitutes a good source of fiber, protein, carbohydrates, and healthy fats, and to differentiate between saturated and unsaturated fats.

Chapter 10. Nutritional Prioritization

Defined health goals can shape your nutritional decisions. For instance, if your aim is to build muscle or improve performance in physical activities, you will need to ensure adequate protein intake. If managing blood sugar levels is your priority, understanding and selecting foods with a low Glycemic Index (GI) will be crucial.

10.1. Creating a Positive Food Environment

Maintaining a conducive food environment goes a long way in supporting healthy food decisions. Keep nutritious foods at hand. Substitute junk snacks with healthier alternatives. Make meal times peaceful and enjoyable.

10.2. Nurturing Food Relationships

The relationship we have with our food is as important as what we eat. Mindful eating can turn every meal into a sensory experience, where we savour each bite, remain aware about the act of eating, appreciate the food and acknowledge the satiety signals which prevents overeating.

10.3. Developing Healthy Habits

Developing habits like regular meal times, eating a balanced breakfast, staying hydrated, consuming moderate portions, and listening to your hunger and satiety signals can significantly enhance your wellness journey.

10.4. Staying Flexible and Adapting

It's crucial to remember that there will be times when sticking to plan might be challenging. Stay flexible, adapt to circumstances, and at the same time, remember your health goals.

In summary, aligning your food choices with your health goals involves understanding your objectives, making informed choices, creating a conducive environment, cultivating a healthy relationship with food, and developing beneficial habits while staying adaptable. As we dive deeper into the following chapters, we will unravel the intricacies of mindful eating and optimal nutrition, arming you with an arsenal of knowledge to help you on your health journey. Get ready to unfold the layers of thoughtfulness, understanding, and attention to find the harmony between your health goals and food choices. Together, let's build a healthier future, meal by meal.

Chapter 11. Understanding and Managing Food Cravings

We've all experienced food cravings - those intense desires for specific foods that can seem impossible to resist. But why do they happen? And how can we manage them to help achieve our health and nutrition goals?

11.1. The Science Behind Food Cravings

Food cravings are driven by a combination of factors including physical needs, brain chemistry, societal influence, and emotional state. Let's take a closer look at how each of these impacts our desire for certain foods.

First, it's important to understand that your body communicates with you through these cravings. Craving salty items, like chips or pretzels, might indicate that your body is low on sodium - an electrolyte necessary for proper body function.

Brain chemistry also plays a significant role in food cravings. Dopamine, a neurotransmitter associated with feelings of pleasure and reward, is released when we eat foods high in fat, sugar, or salt. Over time, our brains can associate these foods with the release of dopamine, leading to cravings.

On top of this, societal influence and the omnipresence of food advertisements can amplify our cravings. It has been shown in numerous studies that repeated exposure to images of high-calorie foods can increase our desire for these items.

Lastly, food can be a source of emotional comfort. Stress, boredom, and sadness are often triggers for food cravings as eating particular foods can lead to quick, albeit temporary, relief from negative emotions. Understanding these emotional triggers is crucial in managing cravings effectively.

11.2. Practical Tips to Manage Food Cravings

Now that we know why food cravings occur, let's explore some strategies to manage them. Here's your guide to mindful eating in the face of cravings.

1. Recognize and Acknowledge Your Cravings

First and foremost, identify when you're having a craving and admit it to yourself, without judgement. This simple act of recognition can distance you from the urge and help you explore why it happened and how to respond.

2. Understand Your Triggers

Jot down when your cravings occur and what's happening at that time. Are you stressed, bored, or sad? Are you really hungry, or are you dehydrated? Recognizing your triggers will help you be proactive in managing your cravings.

3. Opt for Healthier Substitutes

If you're craving something sweet, instead of reaching out for a candy bar, snack on a piece of fruit. If saltiness is what you're after, why not try some lightly salted nuts or popcorn? You get to satisfy your cravings, but in a healthier way.

4. Eat Regular, Balanced Meals

Ensure your meals provide a balance of protein, carbohydrates and healthy fats. A well-rounded meal will leave you feeling satisfied and less likely to have cravings.

5. Stay Hydrated

Sometimes, dehydration disguises itself as hunger. Make sure you're well-hydrated throughout the day; it might reduce your need for snacking.

6. Work Up a Sweat

Exercise plays a dual role - it helps curb cravings and keeps stress at bay. Even a short 15-minute walk can work wonders.

7. Practice Mindful Eating

Savour your food. Take small bites, chew slowly, and appreciate the flavour, texture, and smell. This can help you feel more satisfied and less likely to give in to cravings later.

11.3. Learning from Cravings

Far from being an enemy to combat, food cravings can be an enlightening tool for self-understanding. They provide insight into our nutritional deficiencies, emotional states, and societal conditioning around food. Learning to recognize and manage your food cravings through understanding and mindfulness will aid in establishing a healthy relationship with food. Remember, cravings are natural. It's how we tackle them that makes a difference.

11.4. Conclusion: Journey Towards a Better Relationship with Food

Managing food cravings can indeed be a challenge, but with insight into why we experience them and practical strategies, we can navigate this journey towards healthier eating habits. While it might seem daunting initially, rest assured that every small step brings you closer to maintaining a balanced and nutritious diet. You're embarking on this journey not just for better physical health, but also for a more mindful and enriching relationship with food. It's time to embrace this journey, one craving at a time. It's not about deprivation; it's about making enlightened choices. And remember, this is a gradual transformation - so be patient with yourself. Growth happens bite by bite, day by day.

Chapter 12. Recipes for Health and mindfulness

The omnivores among us are blessed with an almost embarrassingly rich array of foods to choose from. But in life, as in a restaurant, making the right choice isn't always easy. We're here to share recipes that not only promote health but also mindfulness.

12.1. Mindful and Healthful Breakfast Recipes

Did you know that a mindful breakfast can set the tone for your entire day? Here are some recipes that mix nutrition with tranquility:

Avocado Toast with Poached Eggs: Not only a millennial favorite, avocado toast provides healthy fats and antioxidants. For this, you need toasted whole grain bread, avocado mash, poached eggs, salt, and pepper. Spread the avocado, sprinkle some salt and pepper to taste and top with a poached egg. Engage your senses as you savor each bite.

Overnight Oats: If you're always rushing in the morning, prep this the night before. Mix rolled oats, Greek yogurt, chia seeds, a sweetener like honey or agave, and your choice of milk in a mason jar. Let sit overnight in the fridge. The next day, top it with nuts, seeds, or fresh fruits. As you eat, pay attention to these different textures and tastes.

12.2. Lunch Recipes that Energize and Satisfy

If you're looking for a midday meal that will boost your energy and satisfy your hunger, these thoughtful recipes are sure to help:

Quinoa Salad: This gluten-free grain is packed with protein and fiber. Combine cooked and cooled quinoa with vegetables of your choosing, some feta or goat cheese, and a simple olive oil and lemon dressing. Cherish how each forkful delivers different flavors.

Healthy Chicken Wrap: Use a whole wheat tortilla and fill it with grilled chicken, avocado, lettuce, tomatoes, and a light Greek yogurt dressing. Observe the kaleidoscope of colors inside your wrap and appreciate its wholesome goodness.

12.3. Nourishing and Gratifying Dinner Recipes

Evening meals should not only nourish you, but they should also bring you comfort and satisfaction. Here are meals that can help you unwind as your day ends:

Baked Salmon & Veggie Stir-fry: Combine heart-healthy salmon with a stir-fry of your favorite vegetables. Drizzle a bit of olive oil and sprinkle some herbs and spices to taste. The vibrant hues and intricate tastes will engage your senses as you eat mindfully.

Chickpea Curry: Hearty and brimming with flavors. Sauté onions, garlic, and ginger until fragrant. Add in diced tomatoes, chickpeas, coconut milk, and spices like turmeric, cumin, and garam masala. Simmer until infused. Relish the layering of tastes as you mindfully partake in this warm, comforting dish.

12.4. Snacks That Pack a Nutritional Punch

When hunger strikes between meals, these healthful snacks can keep you satisfied:

Apple and Almond Butter: Slice an apple and serve with a side of almond butter. Feel your teeth crunch into the apple and the contrasting creaminess of the almond butter on your tongue.

Greek Yogurt and Berries: Top greek yogurt with your choice of berries - the tanginess of the yogurt coupled with the sweetness of the berries making for an inviting mix of flavors.

With mindful eating, the journey can be just as important, if not more so, than the destination. So as you try these recipes, remember to savor each bite, enjoy each moment and stay focused during your nourishing meals. Listen to your body's signals of fullness, and most importantly, find joy and gratitude in the process of eating.

These recipes aim to provide you not only with food for your body, but food for your mind as well — a feast that aligns your physical and mental wellness goals. So, it's time to grab your apron and embark on this exciting culinary venture towards mindful eating and optimal nutrition. Stay mindful. Stay healthy.

Chapter 13. Grocery Shopping: A New Approach

We've all had those times when we walk into a supermarket on an empty stomach and promptly make a beeline for the cookie aisle. Grocery shopping can be an overwhelming task, but with a bit of planning and a new approach, it can become an enjoyable activity that supports your journey towards mindful eating and optimal nutrition.

13.1. Understand Your Shopping Habits

Before diving into the various strategies for healthy grocery shopping, it's crucial to understand and reflect on your current grocery shopping habits. Everyone has different shopping styles, from impulse buyers who purchase whatever appeals to them at the moment, to methodical shoppers who stick closely to a pre-prepared list. Reflecting on how you shop can help you identify areas for improvement and better tailor your new shopping approach.

13.2. Plan Ahead

Now that we've examined our shopping habits, let's turn our attention to how we can revolutionize our grocery shopping experience. One of the best ways to ensure a mindful shopping experience is to plan ahead. This involves three steps:

- Meal Planning

- Making a Detailed Shopping List

- Researching Store Layouts

Chapter 14. Meal Planning

Creating a meal plan for the week helps to limit unhealthy or impulsive food choices. Include a mix of your favorite meals, new recipes you'd like to try, and simple backup meals for busy days.

Your meal plan should balance macronutrients (protein, fats, and carbohydrates) and include a variety of vegetables, fruits, lean proteins, whole grains and healthy fats. Consider the recommended portion sizes for your nutritional needs, and incorporate foods that host a variety of vitamins, minerals and fiber.

Chapter 15. Detailed Shopping List

Creating a detailed list based on your meal plan ensures you only buy what you need to avoid wastage and extra costs. A good way to structure your list is to categorize items based on their respective department in the store. This not only saves time during shopping, but also limits your exposure to unhealthy food aisles.

Chapter 16. Research Store Layouts

Most supermarkets are designed with the same basic layout. Fresh produce, dairy, meat, and other perishable items are usually located along the periphery, while packaged and processed foods are found in the middle aisles.

Sticking to the outer rim ensures you fill your basket with fresh, whole foods and reduces the temptation to grab unhealthy snacks from the center aisles. If you need items from the middle aisles, try to choose whole grain, low sodium, low sugar options.

16.1. Reading Labels

Understanding food labels is a crucial skill for mindful grocery shopping. Look beyond promotional claims on the front of the package and navigate directly to the nutrition facts panel and ingredient list.

Focus on the serving size and nutrient values first. A package could contain multiple servings, so ensure you're consuming the listed nutrients in the given quantity. Pay close attention to saturated fat, trans fat, sodium, total sugars, proteins, and dietary fiber content.

The ingredient list can reveal a lot about the product's nutritional content. Ingredients are listed in descending order by weight, so the first three ingredients are typically the most abundant. Avoid products where sugar, salt or unhealthy fats like trans or saturated fats are listed in the top three.

16.2. Choosing the Right Produce

Selecting fresh, high-quality produce can be daunting, particularly for seasonal fruits and vegetables, where quality can vary. Here are a few pointers to keep in mind:

- Fruits: Choose fruits that are firm to the touch, have a vibrant color and a fresh smell. Avoid fruits with deep bruises or cuts.

- Vegetables: Choose crisp, vibrant, and firm vegetables. Avoid those with discoloration or soft spots.

- Meat: Choose lean cuts and check for consistent color and firm texture. Avoid meat that has discoloration or an unusual odor.

- Fish: Choose fish that has shiny, metallic skin, and clear eyes. Avoid fish that smells overly fishy, as it may indicate it's not fresh.

16.3. Bring Your Own Bags

As a part of maintaining an eco-friendly lifestyle, consider bringing your reusable shopping bags. They're not only a mindful choice for the environment but also help you reevaluate your purchases as you fill up your bags.

By adopting these strategies, grocery shopping will cease to be a mundane chore and transform into a delightful, health-empowering journey instead. It's a powerful step in transforming your relationship with food and steering your life towards better health and wellness.

Chapter 17. The Confluence of Fitness and Nutrition

An understanding of the critical relationship between fitness and nutrition paves the way to achieving a balanced lifestyle. Both are harmoniously intertwined, with one playing a significant role in supporting and augmenting the other. This synergistic effect translates to better health, increased immunity, enhanced physical performance, improved mental focus, and heightened emotional wellbeing.

17.1. The Science Behind Fitness and Nutrition

Fitness and nutrition have a reciprocal relationship. A nutrient-dense diet provides the necessary energy to engage in physical activities, while regular exercise aids in efficiently processing the nutrients consumed. Together, they work as a powerful team, extolling remarkable benefits on health and wellbeing.

Energy balance is one fundamental aspect mediated by the marriage of fitness and nutrition. Calories burned through physical activity should be balanced by calories consumed through diet to maintain a healthy weight. An imbalance in this equation can result in weight gain or loss, both of which can pose challenges to overall health.

On a cellular level, exercise stimulates the production of mitochondria, the powerhouses of cells, for energy expenditure. An optimal nutrition further supports these tiny organelles to function more effectively. Protein-rich foods aid in muscle repair and growth after a workout, carbohydrates provide fuel for endurance activities, and healthy fats assist with hormone production and inflammation control.

17.2. Nutrients and Their Role in Fitness

Nutrition plays a pivotal role in enhancing physical fitness, with different nutrients serving distinct purposes. Dietary proteins, carbohydrates, and fats serve as primary fuel sources, dietary fiber aids in digestion, and vitamins and minerals perform various roles from fostering bone health to boosting the immune system.

Proteins, for instance, are the building blocks of muscle tissue. They aid in repairing the micro-tears caused in muscles during strenuous exercise. Carbohydrates, on the other hand, are the body's preferred energy source, fueling everything from minor activities like walking to major tasks like weightlifting. Lastly, dietary fat, though often perceived negatively, is necessary for optimal health. It provides energy, aids in nutrient absorption, and is vital for hormone production.

17.3. Exercise: A Helpful Ally in Nutrition Digestion

Exercise offers myriad benefits, including promoting efficient digestion and absorption of food, thus increasing the nutritional value intake. It stimulates the muscles in the gastrointestinal tract, which helps move food more efficiently through your system and facilitates better absorption of nutrients.

Moreover, exercise aids in maintaining a healthy metabolism, which consequently enhances the body's ability to process food effectively. Regular physical activity can help manage blood sugar levels, reducing the risk of developing type 2 diabetes. Besides, it assists in managing weight by burning off extra calories, thus preventing obesity, a leading cause of many health issues.

17.4. Dietary Strategies for Exercise

What, when, and how much to eat matter when planning an exercise regime. It's crucial to nourish the body with a balanced plate featuring proteins, carbs, and fats.

Before exercise, a meal or snack rich in carbohydrates can provide the necessary glucose for energy. During longer duration activities, maintaining hydration and easy-to-digest carbohydrates can prevent fatigue. Post-exercise, a balanced meal with adequate protein and carbs supports muscle recovery and replenishes energy stores.

Hydration is also pivotal in fitness. Dehydration can dramatically affect performance and potentially lead to overheating and other health risks. It is recommended to stay hydrated before, during, and after exercise to maintain fluid balance.

17.5. Designing a Balanced Diet and Fitness Regime

Designing a fitness regime and nutrition plan that work in harmony can be daunting. It's crucial to tailor the approach to individual needs, considering age, sex, weight, height, and physical activity level.

Strive for a rich, diverse diet abundant in fruits, vegetables, lean proteins, healthy fats, whole grains, and fiber. Subsequently, integrate physical activity, preferably a mix of cardiovascular workouts, strength training, and flexibility exercises, into the daily routine. Keep in mind that nutritional needs would escalate with the increase in physical activity.

Adopting a mindful approach to eating can also contribute towards achieving fitness goals. Paying close attention to hunger and satiety cues can help regulate food intake and prevent overeating.

Remember, a well-rounded approach to fitness and nutrition doesn't just involve what you eat or how much you exercise. It also includes good sleep habits and stress management, contributing to improved recovery and overall wellbeing.

Embarking on the journey towards a harmonious blend of fitness and nutrition might seem complex, but the resulting health and wellness benefits are beyond rewarding. By nurturing these co-dependent realms, you are setting the foundation for a vibrant life, pulsating with health and vitality.

Chapter 18. Family and Mindful Eating: A Shared Journey

Understanding the role of family in our food habits is paramount to adopting a more mindful eating approach. As we delve into the depths of this subject, we'll explore the influences of familial tradition, societal norms, and individual spaces within a family unit.

18.1. The Familiarity of Food in Family Life

Food is as much a cultural language as it is a requirement of our biological systems. In numerous cultures, family meals hold sacred significance. They are the very threads that weave together the tapestry of love, shared history, and belonging in a family. More often than not, our dietary habits, our food preferences, and even our attitudes toward eating are deeply embedded in our family history.

Understanding this dynamic is the first step toward mindful eating. From early childhood, we learn our food behaviors from observing and imitating our families. If the family habit is rushing through meals, not paying attention to what's on the plate, or eating in an emotionally charged atmosphere, these behaviors tend to be replicated throughout our lives, forming an almost indistinguishable part of our identities.

Recognizing and acknowledging these patterns is the first step to making a positive shift toward mindful eating.

18.2. Breaking the Chain: Reconditioning Family Food Habits

The act of breaking familial food habits does not imply turning one's back on years of tradition. Instead, it means recognizing the parts of these traditions that may not be serving us well. This could be anything from consuming unhealthy amounts of a specific food type, mindlessly snacking, or eating under stress.

Once recognized, we can set about making collective changes to these habits. Start by introducing mindful eating practices at meals: focusing solely on the meal, banishing distractions, eating slowly, and creating an atmosphere of enjoyment and appreciation for the food on the table. The change may not come overnight, but with persistence, new habits can become a natural part of your family's mealtime tradition.

18.3. Developing a Collective Relationship with Food: Mindfulness for All

Devoting time and effort to change the way your family approaches food may initially seem daunting, but the resulting benefits are immense. Mindful eating promotes healthier food choices and a healthier relationship with food by centering around the experience of eating, and emphasizing quality over quantity.

Begin small. Make it a practice to sit together at meals with no distractions. Encourage everyone to taste their food fully, to note the sensation of chewing, and the taste, texture, and aroma of different ingredients. Talk about where the food comes from and show appreciation for the nourishment it provides.

Remember, it is about making a journey together as a family towards healthier habits that include not just what you eat, but how, why and when you eat as well.

18.4. The Mindful Kitchen: Where Change Begins

As an extension of mindful eating, adopting mindfulness in the kitchen adds a new dimension to your relationship with food. From the moment you decide on a meal, the process of preparing it, the act of cooking, to the final plating, and cleaning up - each step provides an opportunity for mindfulness.

Involve family members in kitchen tasks to shift the perspective on food preparation from a choresome duty to a joy-filled, shared activity. Celebrate the colors, textures, and indeed, the life within different foods. Take note of the origins of ingredients, each with its own journey that led it to your kitchen. Discover the connection with the world around in the simple act of preparing a meal.

Over time, even these conscious changes can result in a deeper respect for food, a greater awareness of one's eating habits, and a heightened sense of responsibility towards reducing food waste, creating a healthier lifestyle for the entire family.

In conclusion, the role of the family is imperative in fostering mindful eating habits. What may seem like a challenge in the beginning grows into a shared journey of awareness and appreciation for the food we consume. Start small, have patience, and you'll soon discover that the journey towards mindful eating is a delicious one, and a journey best made together.

Chapter 19. Sustaining Your Nutrition Goals: Tips and Tricks

Achieving your nutrition goals requires commitment, determination, consistency, and astute understanding of food and its implications on your health. Yet, even with these prerequisites in place, sustaining such changes over the long term can be challenging. This chapter delves into the intricacies of sustaining your nutrition goals, offering a comprehensive, well-rounded collection of tips and tricks.

19.1. Know Your Why

Recognizing the motives behind your pursuit of a healthier diet is crucial. Is it a medical necessity, weight management, enhanced physical performance, or mere curiosity? Defining your 'why' will serve as a motivational compass, continuously pointing you towards your goal, even in the face of temptation.

19.2. Set Clear, Achievable Goals

Goals that are too ambitious or vague often lead to frustration and eventual abandonment of one's pursuit. Remember, Rome was not built in a day. Your nutrition goals should challenge you, but also feel achievable and realistic. Start small, perhaps by incorporating more vegetables into your diet or reducing your sugar intake, and gradually build upon these steps to mount a larger change.

19.3. Understand Your Food

Equip yourself with knowledge about food itself. Understanding the macronutrients (proteins, fats, carbohydrates), micronutrients (vitamins, minerals), their roles, sources, and recommended daily allowances can empower you in constructing a balanced dietary regime.

19.4. Keep Up with Regular Health Checkups

Regular health checkups provide tangible evidence of your nutritional endeavor's impact. Tracking parameters related to nutrition – blood lipid profile, glucose levels, vitamin levels – can reinforce your commitment to maintaining nutritional changes.

19.5. Meal Planning and Prepping

Planning meals ahead can reduce impulsive, unhealthy food choices. Dedicate a specific day of the week to meal planning, grocery shopping, and basic preparation. This approach saves time and ensures you are well-stocked with healthful options.

19.6. Savor The Flavor

Eating healthily does not mean abandoning taste. Explore herbs, spices, and different cooking methods to add diversity and flavor to your meals. Remember, food that is enjoyable is much easier to sustain in a diet.

19.7. Listen to Your Body

Learn to recognize genuine hunger, thirst, and satiety cues. Eat when you're truly hungry, not just bored or stressed. Make hydration a priority, and stop eating when satisfied, not just when your plate is empty.

19.8. Practice Portion Control

Be mindful of portion sizes. Even the healthiest of foods, when consumed in excess, can derail your nutrition goals. Learn to estimate portions accurately and stick to recommended serving sizes.

19.9. Physical Activity

Regular physical activity complements your nutrition goals, helping enhance the efficiency of nutrient utilization, and maintaining an energy balance. Choose an activity that you enjoy and can adhere to in the long run.

19.10. Cultivate a Positive Mindset

Maintaining a positive mindset and associating joy with your new dietary habits can prove an incredibly strong reinforcing tool. Celebrate each successful step towards your nutrition goal, however small.

19.11. Don't Beat Yourself Up Over a Slip-Up

Everyone has instances where they fall off the wagon. Instead of berating yourself, accept the mishap as a part of the journey. Reflect on what led to the slip-up, and use that insight to fortify your commitment.

19.12. Get Support

A support system can significantly aid your journey towards sustained nutrition goals. It could be family, friends, like-minded communities, or professional health coaches. Share your goals with them, and seek their encouragement and assistance.

19.13. Keep Educating Yourself

With the dynamic realm of nutrition, new research and findings emerge frequently. Keeping abreast with this knowledge can further refine your dietary habits and reinforce your commitment.

19.14. Adapt and Modify

It's okay to modify your goals as you progress. If you observe that a certain strategy is not working for you, or if your health parameters have changed, adapt and tweak your goals accordingly. Flexibility is key for long-term sustainability.

As you navigate through your nutritional journey, these tips and tricks can serve as your roadmap, ensuring you stay on the path, adapt where necessary, and maintain the changes successfully. Falling and failing are merely part of the journey, but with resilience, resolve, and the right resources, you can successfully sustain your new nutrition habits, moving towards optimal health and wellness.

Chapter 20. Moving Forward: An Eternally Nutritious Tomorrow

In the pursuit of a healthier future, our focus turns towards sustainability, not just in terms of food sources but building habits that stand the test of time. It is not only about losing those extra pounds temporarily or momentarily eliminating certain diseases, better eating ought to be an enduring commitment to ourselves.

20.1. Understanding Sustainable Eating Habits

Preceding the beginning of making changes, we must understand what it means to have sustainable eating habits. Essentially this refers to those patterns of consumption which, once established, can be maintained over a lifetime. This is not only beneficial to your health but also factors into global sustainability, as it means leaning towards organic, locally sourced and seasonal food, and away from processed foods that are high in sugars, salt, and unhealthy fats. Sustainable eating habits are not a fad diet; they require no drastic culinary overhauls, but a slow, mindful transition is beneficial to leading a healthier lifestyle.

Sustainable eating is anchored on the tenet that 'good food' nourishes the body, satiates the mind, and respects our planet. There are a few pillars -

1) Locally sourced food: Food grown close to home tends to be fresher, contain fewer chemicals, and support local economies. 2) Seasonal food: Seasonal eating encourages diversification of diet and reduces dependence on far-away food sources. 3) Minimal food

wastage: By carefully planning meals and portions. 4) Balanced Diet: Ensure that the meals you prepare cater to all the nutrient needs of your body.

20.2. Building Lasting Habits

Building sustainable, healthy habits is the key to achieving nutritional wellness, but the process can be challenging. Breaking down old, unhealthy patterns and replacing them with new, wholesome ones requires time, patience, and a few strategically chosen steps.

1) Start small: Rather than trying to modify your entire diet in one go, begin by introducing small changes such as switching to whole grains or adding more fruits and vegetables to your meals.

2) Personalize your diet: Since everyone's nutrient requirements differ, there is no one-size-fits-all diet plan. Your sustainable diet should be tailored to your unique needs, preferences, and lifestyle.

3) Think of intention, not restrictions: Instead of seeing your health journey as a series of banning certain types of food, focus on incorporating more healthy options.

20.3. Meeting Nutritional Needs Sustainably: Practical Tips

Once the broad principles are clear, let's delve into the specifics of how we can meet our nutritional needs in a sustainable way.

1) Keep hydrated: Drink enough water every day to keep the body functioning at its optimum.

2) Incorporate proteins: Ensure adequate intake of protein in every meal which aids in growth and repair.

3) Prioritize fiber: High-fiber foods like whole grains, fruits, and vegetables promote feelings of fullness, keeps your gut healthy and manages blood sugar levels.

4) Healthy fats are your friend: Choose healthy fats from plant sources like avocados, nuts, seeds and olive oil.

5) Reduce added sugars: Mindful reduction in the consumption of high sugar foods and beverages can have a significant impact on your overall health.

By following these tips, and adapting them to your personal needs, maintaining sustainable healthy eating habits will become a part of your day-to-day life.

20.4. The Journey Ahead

As this chapter guides you towards sustainable eating habits, remember that change isn't a switch to be flipped but a dial to be turned. The journey towards healthy eating is not always linear. There will be victories, and there will be missteps – but even the missteps are valuable, as they provide us with the opportunity to learn and make more informed decisions moving forward.

Let this 'Eternally Nutritious Tomorrow' be the goal that shapes your food choices. Every bite should be a step closer to health, a step closer to sustainability and one more victory in the journey towards a balanced, nutritional lifestyle. It's time that we not just eat, but nourish ourselves. For that is the path towards not just existent but vibrant living, where our bodies are not just surviving but thriving. In the grand orchestra of life, let mindful, nutritious eating be the sweet melody that keeps us dancing to the symphony of health and happiness.

And with that, we continue to explore the realm of mindful eating and optimal nutrition, charting our path into a healthier, happier, and more vibrant tomorrow. Let's embrace this journey towards a better future, one nourishing meal at a time.